NATIONAL MEDICAL ADVISORY COMMITTEE

The Management of Anxiety and Insomnia

A Report by the National Medical Advisory Committee

June 1994

HMSO: EDINBURGH

First published 1994

ISBN 0 11 495274 4

Terms of Reference

"To review the current position on the prescribing of anxiolytics and hypnotics and to make recommendations for change with guidelines which include the need to minimise abuse."

FOREWORD

This report was prepared by a multidisciplinary Working Group set up by the National Medical Advisory Committee and chaired by Dr J D Gilleghan, an Edinburgh general practitioner. It is explicitly intended to help Scottish doctors reduce their prescribing, particularly long-term prescribing, of benzodiazepines and other hypnotic and anxiolytic drugs, while at the same time meeting the needs of their patients for relief from anxiety, tension and insomnia. A great deal of attention has been given to the detailed layout of the report, particularly to the provision of clear, practical advice on the use of psychological and other non-pharmacological treatments for anxiety and insomnia, and on strategies for the management of benzodiazepine withdrawal.

Although the number of prescriptions issued in Scotland for anxiolytics and hypnotics has fallen by 32% in the last decade over 2.4 million prescriptions were still issued for these drugs in 1992, one for every other man, woman and child in the country. There are also substantial differences in prescribing levels in different Health Board areas.

There are two important reasons for reducing the prescribing of anxiolytics and hypnotics. Most, if not all, are habit forming and their use for longer than a few weeks easily leads to dependence. Drug misuse is also a major and increasing problem in Scotland. Temazepam, a widely prescribed benzodiazepine, is one of the most important of these misused drugs and evidence from many sources suggests that NHS prescriptions are the main source of supply.

For both these reasons this Report is welcomed by The Scottish Office Home and Health Department.

R E KENDELL
Chief Medical Officer

CONTENTS

EXECUTIVE SUMMARY

This Report has been prompted by the evidence that temazepam has become a major drug of misuse in Scotland and the recent investigation by the Scottish Affairs Committee into Drug Abuse.

The original remit placed emphasis upon the need to reduce the prescribing of anxiolytics and hypnotics but because the use of non-drug strategies is so important, the Working Group was encouraged to examine its remit from a wider perspective as reflected in the title of the Report.

The Report is designed to help doctors to look more critically at benzodiazepine prescribing and provides information and advice on how to continue to reduce levels of prescribing over time.

The Report highlights some of the problems encountered in current practice in the hospital and the community and cites evidence received from the Home Office Drugs Inspectorate that most misused benzodiazepines are obtained on prescription.

The Report suggests practical ways in which some of the problems can be addressed, laying particular emphasis on the development of guidelines designed to reduce the level of prescribing, and encourages the use of non-drug management. Sample letters together with simple measures to combat anxiety and insomnia are included in the text and may be freely adapted for local use.

I INTRODUCTION

1. The management of anxiety and insomnia, with undue reliance on the prescribing of anxiolytics and hypnotics, is currently the subject of much public and professional concern.

Historical Perspective

2. Until about 30 years ago, most symptoms of anxiety and insomnia, when treated at all, were treated with barbiturate drugs. In the 1960s these drugs were quickly supplanted by benzodiazepines which had fewer side-effects and were much less dangerous than barbiturates in overdosage. Benzodiazepines are now the most commonly used anxiolytics and hypnotics, and barbiturates are no longer recommended for these purposes.

3. In 1988, the Committee on Safety of Medicines declared that the use of benzodiazepines should be reduced as dependence was becoming the subject of increasing concern.

4. The scale of benzodiazepine prescribing should not be underestimated. In 1982, there were 25 benzodiazepines on the world market. These were marketed under 340 brand names and manufactured in 13 countries. In the UK, at that time, between 18 and 20 million prescriptions were issued for tranquillisers and approximately 14 million prescriptions for hypnotics. Although the level of benzodiazepine prescribing remains very high in Scotland, there has been a steady decline in recent years. Table I shows an overall reduction in the past ten years by around one third.

5. Differentials which exist in the level of prescribing of benzodiazepines between Scottish Health Boards are shown in Table II. It is hoped that the considerable reductions achieved in some Health Board areas will soon be attained by all.

Reasons for Review

6. The need for this review has been prompted by the evidence that temazepam has become a major drug of misuse in Scotland, the current investigation by the Scottish Affairs Committee into Drug Abuse, and professional and public concern over the addictive potential of anxiolytics and hypnotics. It is recognised that the problem in Scotland with benzodiazepines as drugs of misuse is greater than in other parts of the UK.

Aim of the Report

7. The aim of this report is to encourage a shift towards the use, where appropriate, of the non-drug management of anxiety and insomnia. It is hoped to continue the reduction of the prescribing of anxiolytics and hypnotics through the use of guidelines on prescribing in hospitals and in the community.

TABLE I: NUMBER OF PRESCRIPTIONS ISSUED PER YEAR FOR ANXIOLYTICS AND HYPNOTICS IN SCOTLAND

1982	3,546,000
1983	3,448,000
1984	3,377,000
1985	3,129,000
1986	3,049,000
1987	3,317,000
1988	3,146,000
1989	2,750,000
1990	2,543,000
1991	2,521,000
1992	2,402,000

Source: Management Information and Research Centre, Pharmacy Practice Division.

TABLE II: TOTAL BENZODIAZEPINE PRESCRIBING: SCOTLAND AND SCOTTISH HEALTH BOARDS: JULY TO SEPTEMBER 1993

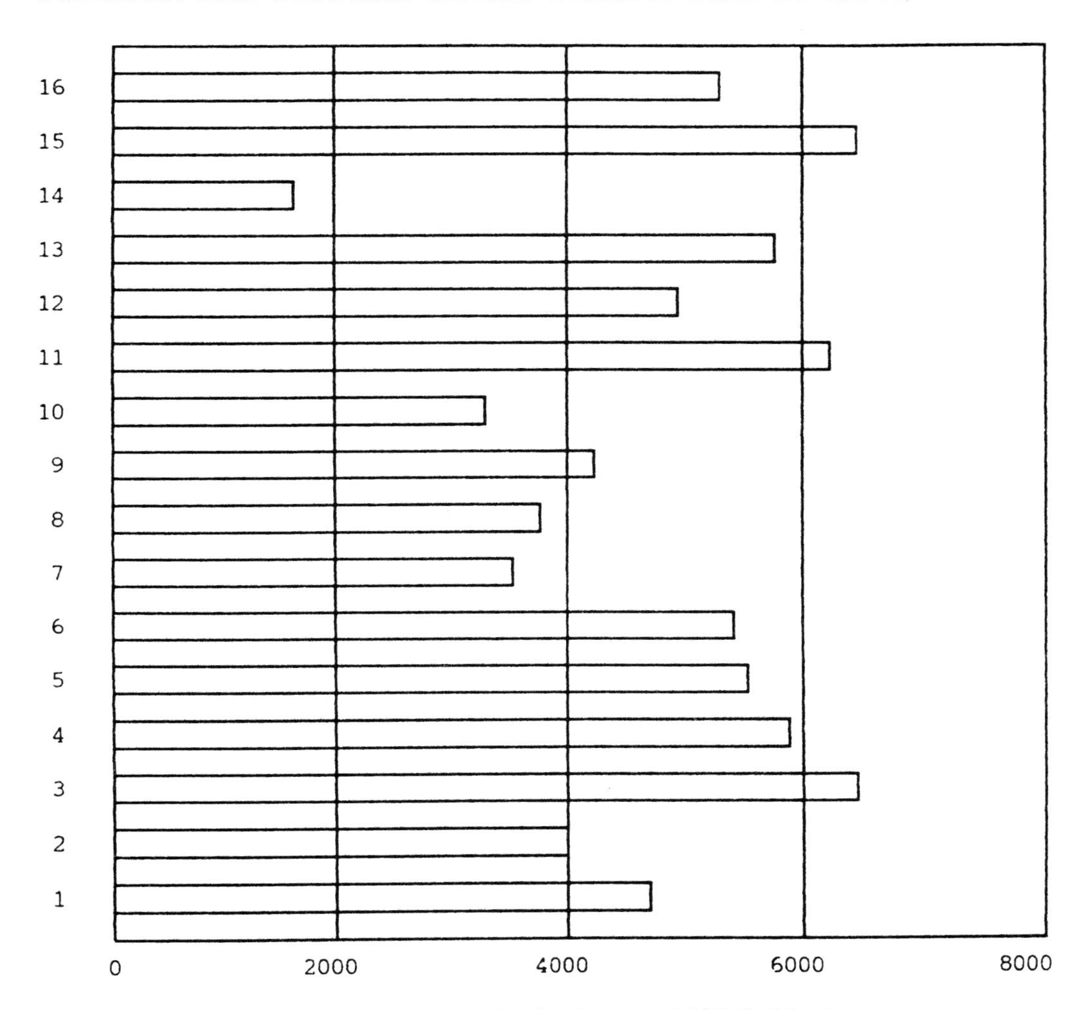

5 mg Diazepam Equivalents per 1000 Patients

1	Borders	9	Western Isles
2	Fife	10	Orkney
3	Lanarkshire	11	Forth Valley
4	Tayside	12	Lothian
5	Argyll and Clyde	13	Dumfries and Galloway
6	Greater Glasgow	14	Shetland
7	Highland	15	Ayrshire and Arran
8	Grampian	16	Scotland

Source: Pharmacy Practice Division

II THE MANAGEMENT OF ANXIETY AND INSOMNIA

Introduction

8. Patients presenting with anxiety or insomnia should be assessed and diagnosed; emotional and practical problems need to be addressed and a range of treatment options considered.

9. The following algorithm sets out the different stages that need to be followed in the management process. Wherever possible, non-drug strategies should be considered for the management of anxiety or insomnia.

NON-DRUG MANAGEMENT

10. Psychological treatments can provide an effective form of therapy for patients suffering from insomnia and patients with acute reactions to stress, generalised anxiety disorder, agoraphobia and panic disorders. The main forms of treatment are self-monitoring, applied relaxation - including hypnotherapy - counselling, anxiety management, behavioural therapy and cognitive therapy.

11. It is suggested that many of these non-drug treatments can be introduced into the general practice consultation. Specialist referral is indicated only where the patient clearly presents with a severe complex problem, or where further help is required to promote a more complete therapeutic response. The implementation of such psychological treatments need not be time-consuming when it is supplemented by written material to reinforce advice from the consultation. Many patients appreciate this level of involvement in addressing their own situation.

12. All patients presenting with anxiety and insomnia require assessment and self-monitoring. Self-monitoring through the use of a behavioural diary or sleep diary is not only a good test of patient motivation but also a means of giving the patient a shared sense of responsibility for his or her health. Examples of both types of diary are given in this section and may be freely copied or adapted for local use.

MANAGEMENT OF ANXIETY AND INSOMNIA

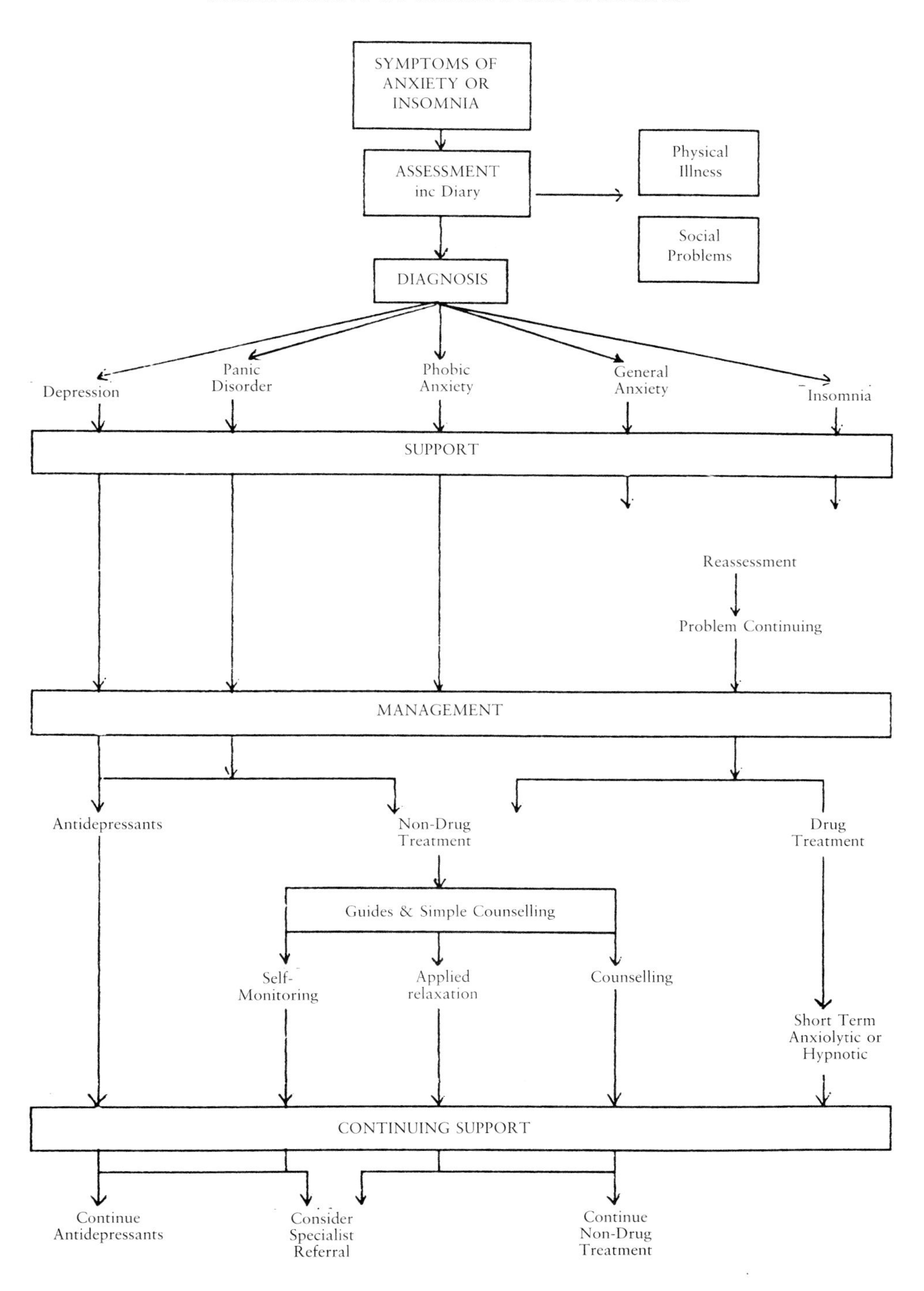

13. Applied relaxation, hypnosis and self-hypnosis, can be used as a general technique for coping with anxiety or insomnia. Audio-tapes or written material can supplement counselling to assist the patient to develop helpful strategies. A Good Sleep Guide and Good Relaxation Guide are presented in this report and both may be freely copied or adapted for local use.

14. Counselling can be an appropriate form of treatment for mild symptoms of anxiety where the origins of the problem are obvious. This involves discussion with the patient, and sometimes the patient's family, in order to help the patient to come to terms with symptoms of anxiety and to resolve any life problems. Referral, when required, should be to a trained counsellor.

15. Educational approaches may be advantageous when there is a need to treat large numbers of patients. General practitioners should consider that feasibility of introducing clinics or courses on anxiety management skills run by, for example, clinical psychologists, community psychiatric nurses or non-statutory agencies. Running a course enables several patients to be seen at once. The educational context encourages participation and mutual support. Responsibility for attendance gives the patient a personal sense of accountability for his or her health.

16. It is envisaged that all these non-drug treatments can be managed in the general practice consultation. However, some patients may require specialised treatment. This can be provided by a clinical psychologist or other suitably trained professionals. Behavioural therapy can help patients to learn how to replace unhelpful ways of coping, such as the deliberate avoidance of situations that provoke anxiety, with helpful ones. The emphasis is placed on tackling the factors that maintain the disorder as opposed to those that have caused it. Cognitive therapy can be of assistance in teaching the patient how to control anxiety by learning to identify, challenge and alter long-established false assumptions that exacerbate or prolong anxiety.

BEHAVIOURAL DIARY

A typical behaviour diary:

Day and Date	Time	Place and Situation	Severity (0- 0)

Example:

BEHAVIOURAL DIARY - ANXIETY

Day and Date	Time	Place and Situation	Severity (0- 0)
Monday 11th	9pm	Home. Watching TV.	7
Tuesday 12th	7am	Home. Shaving.	7
Wednesday 13th	11am 4pm	Walking to shops Home. Visitor arrived unexpectedly	8

SLEEP DIARY

Name: .... Week beginning: ....

MEASURING THE PATTERN OF YOUR SLEEP

	Day 1	Day 2	Day 3	Day 4	Day 5	Day 6	Day 7
1. At what time did you get up this morning?							
2. At what time did you go to your bed last night?							
3. How long did it take you to fall asleep (mins)?							
4. How many times did you wake up during the night?							
5. How long were you awake <u>during</u> the night (in total)?							
6. About how long did you sleep altogether (hours/mins)?							
7. How much alcohol did you take last night?							
8. How many sleeping pills did you take to help you sleep?							

MEASURING THE QUALITY OF YOUR SLEEP

	Day 1	Day 2	Day 3	Day 4	Day 5	Day 6	Day 7
1. How well do you feel this morning? 0 not at all, 1, 2 moderately, 3, 4 very							
2. How enjoyable was your sleep last night? 0 not at all, 1, 2 moderately, 3, 4 very							
3. How mentally alert were you in bed last night? 0 not at all, 1, 2 moderately, 3, 4 very							
4. How physically tense were you in bed last night? 0 not at all, 1, 2 moderately, 3, 4 very							

THE GOOD SLEEP GUIDE

DURING THE EVENING

1. Put the day to rest. Think it through. Tie up "loose ends" in your mind and plan ahead. A notebook may help.
2. Take some light exercise early in the evening. Generally try to keep yourself fit.
3. Wind down during the course of the evening. Do not do anything that is mentally demanding within 90 minutes of bedtime.
4. Do not sleep or doze in the armchair. Keep your sleep for bedtime.
5. Do not drink too much coffee or tea and only have a light snack for supper. Do not drink alcohol to aid your sleep - it usually upsets sleep.
6. Make sure your bed and bedroom are comfortable - not too cold and not too warm.

AT BEDTIME

1. Go to bed when you are "sleepy tired" and not before.
2. Do not read or watch TV in bed. Keep these activities for another room.
3. Set the alarm for the same time every day - 7 days a week, at least until your sleep pattern settles down.
4. Put the light out when you get into bed.
5. Let yourself relax and tell yourself that "sleep will come when it`s ready". Enjoy relaxing even if you don`t at first fall asleep.
6. Do not try to fall asleep. Sleep is not something you can switch on deliberately but if you try to switch it on you can switch it off!

IF YOU HAVE PROBLEMS GETTING TO SLEEP

1. Remember that sleep problems are quite common and they are not as damaging as you might think. Try not to get upset or frustrated.

2. If you are awake in bed for more than 20 minutes then get up and go into another room.

3. Do something relaxing for a while and don`t worry about tomorrow. People usually cope quite well even after a sleepless night.

4. Go back to bed when you feel "sleepy tired".

5. Remember the tips from the section above and use them again.

6. A good sleep pattern may take a number of weeks to establish. Be confident that you will achieve this in the end by working through the "GOOD SLEEP GUIDE"!

This guide has been adapted from material originally prepared by Dr Colin Espie.

THE GOOD RELAXATION GUIDE

DEALING WITH PHYSICAL TENSION

1. Value times of relaxation. Think of them as essentials not extras. Give relaxation some of your best time not just what's left over.

2. Build relaxing things into your lifestyle every day and take your time. Don't rush. Don't try too hard.

3. Learn a relaxation routine, but don't expect to learn without practice.

4. There are many relaxation routines available, especially on audio tape. These help you to reduce muscle tension and to learn how to use your breathing to help you relax.

5. Tension can show in many different ways - aches, stiffness, heart racing, perspiration, stomach churning etc. Don't be worried about this.

6. Keep fit. Physical exercise, such as a regular brisk walk or a swim, can help to relieve tension.

DEALING WITH WORRY

1. Accept that worry can be normal and that it can be useful. Some people worry more than others but everyone worries sometimes.

2. Write down your concerns. Decide which ones are more important by rating each out of ten.

3. Work out a plan of action for each problem.

4. Share your worries. Your friends or your general practitioner can give you helpful advice.

5. Doing crosswords, reading, taking up a hobby or an interest can all keep your mind active and positive. You can block out worrying thoughts by mentally repeating a comforting phrase.

6. Practice enjoying quiet moments, eg sitting listening to relaxing music. Allow your mind to wander and try to picture yourself in pleasant, enjoyable situations.

DEALING WITH DIFFICULT SITUATIONS

1. Try to build up your confidence. Try not to avoid circumstances where you feel more anxious. A step by step approach is best to help you face things and places which make you feel tense. Regular practice will help you to overcome your anxiety.

2. Make a written plan and decide how you are going to deal with difficult situations.

3. Reward yourself for your successes. Tell others. We all need encouragement.

4. Your symptoms may return as you face up to difficult situations. Keep trying and they should become less troublesome as your confidence grows.

5. Everyone has good days and bad days. Expect to have more good days as time goes on.

6. Try to put together a programme based on all of the elements in "The Good Relaxation Guide" that will meet the needs of your particular situation. Remember that expert guidance and advice is available if you need further help.

This guide has been adapted from material originally prepared by Dr Colin Espie.

DRUG MANAGEMENT

17. Most anxiety states are transient. Treatment with benzodiazepines may occasionally be indicated for a short time.

18. All benzodiazepines carry a potential risk of dependence which means that wherever possible a non-drug strategy should be the preferred line of treatment. All patients should be advised of the risks and benefits of drug treatment.

19. Both longer and shorter acting benzodiazepines appear to possess the potential for dependence but benzodiazepines with shorter half lives have an increased tendency to lead to a withdrawal syndrome. Longer-acting benzodiazepines may lead to accumulation.

HALF-LIFE OF BENZODIAZEPINES IN CURRENT USE IN THE NHS

Drug	Half-life (Hours)	Duration of Action
Chlordiazepoxide	5-30	Long
Diazepam	24-48 (48-120 for active metabolite)	Long
Loprazolam	4-15	Short
Lorazepam	10-20	Short
Lormetazepam	12	Short
Nitrazepam	24	Long
Oxazepam	6-20	Short
Temazepam	8-15	Short
Clonazepam	20-40	Long
Clobazam	24	Long
Midazolam	2-7	Very Short

20. The short-acting drugs oxazepam and lorazepam are frequently associated with withdrawal symptoms. These drugs are not recommended for general use.

21. During the day, a longer acting benzodiazepine, (preferably diazepam), may be considered for the short-term relief of anxiety that is severe. Treatment should initially be limited to one to four weeks.

22. Benzodiazepines should never be prescribed for insomnia without a careful exploration of the aetiology. At nights, shorter acting benzodiazepines (temazepam, lormetazepam, loprazolam) are best, used occasionally rather than regularly.

23. Patients presenting with depression should usually be treated with an antidepressant drug but, in those who are agitated as part of the depression, a sedative antidepressant is preferable to the concomitant use of a benzodiazepine.

24. When attempting to avoid using anxiolytics and hypnotics, the substitution of antidepressants and antipsychotic drugs should be avoided, unless clearly indicated.

25. The prescribing of benzodiazepines should be kept to a minimum, be reviewed on a regular basis and discontinued as soon as possible.

Prescribing in Hospital

26. There should be agreed local guidelines on the prescribing of benzodiazepines, which should conform to the standards published in the British National Formulary. Some wards and units already have prescribing protocols to reduce the use of benzodiazepines. Pharmacists play a valuable role in the joint production of such protocols and the monitoring of their use.

27. A full drug history should be taken on admission.

28. Regular users, particularly the elderly, should not have their medication suddenly withdrawn.

29. Benzodiazepines should not be prescribed for patients who were not taking them prior to admission unless there are strong and genuine indications.

30. Medical staff and/or pharmacy staff should review any patient taking benzodiazepines whilst in hospital and also prior to discharge. The patient`s general practitioner should be informed of action taken.

Prescribing in the Community

31. Many general practitioners are increasingly aware of the problems which arise from benzodiazepine prescribing and are actively addressing them. Much of the long-term prescribing of benzodiazepines was initiated before the Committee on Safety of Medicines` warning in 1988. Since then, the side-effects of benzodiazepines and the problem of dependence have become clearly defined and it is now acknowledged that long-term prescribing is not good practice.

32. Most general practitioners take time to explore the non-pharmacological alternatives to benzodiazepine prescribing for minor psychological disorders and more should be encouraged to do so.

33. In many practices, general practitioners take time to review patients who are on benzodiazepines, inform them of the potential for dependence and offer them practical help and support in the management of withdrawal.

34. Patients receiving their medicines on repeat prescribing systems are not always subject to regular review, nor are they always reminded of the potential dangers associated with continued use.

35. Where care is being shared with a consultant, changes in medication by one doctor may not be communicated to the other, with resultant confusion.

36. Patients taking benzodiazepines at the time of discharge from hospital sometimes have their prescriptions continued by their general practitioner in the absence of information from the hospital.

37. Every general practice should develop guidelines on the prescribing of anxiolytics and hypnotics. A prescribing policy ensures uniformity of prescribing among partners and also encourages good practice.

38. Lay carers at home and professional carers in residential and nursing homes for the elderly, the disabled or those with learning difficulties, should be provided with education on the importance of normal sleeping and waking patterns, and the requirement for daytime stimulation to promote sleep. An information sheet is reproduced at the end of this section, which may be adapted for local use.

39. Withdrawal programmes should be offered to, and agreed with, patients whenever possible, otherwise patients should be regularly reviewed.

40. Drug misuse agencies, community pharmacists and primary care services should develop a co-ordinated strategy for the management of benzodiazepine misuse. There is a need, in service provision, to recognise the important differences between drug misusers and patients who may become dependent upon benzodiazepines prescribed at normal doses.

HELP WITH SLEEP: INFORMATION FOR CARERS

1. Older people need less sleep at night, particularly if they doze during the day.

2. It is important to have a set time for getting up. The time for going to bed can be more flexible.

3. It is normal for older people to awaken several times during the night. This is not harmful. Being awake does not necessarily mean that the individual is distressed. Resting in bed is almost as good as sleeping.

4. A good night's sleep may follow a sleepless night, without the need to resort to a sleeping pill.

5. Physical symptoms, especially pain, which disturb sleep should be treated in their own right.

6. The doctor should be alerted to symptoms of anxiety or depression.

7. A range of activities should be encouraged in order to maintain alertness and interest in life.

8. Sleeping pills are addictive. They should only be used on occasions when they are really needed.

9. Sleeping pills can have "hangover" effects the next day causing difficulty with concentration, dizziness, drowsiness, and falls.

10. As a carer, you should feel able to discuss your own feelings with the doctor. You are entitled to periods of respite care to enable you to have a much-needed break!

Patient Information and Education

41. In the community, general practitioners and pharmacists are often in the best position to offer professional advice to patients on medication but patients are often reluctant to ask questions because of a lack of self-confidence or a general perception that professionals lack time.

42. Information that patients require is often very straightforward but there is always the danger that the information given may be insufficient or forgotten after the event. Information which is communicated in a positive manner, and reinforced by the community pharmacist, can improve patient compliance and act as a stimulus to help the patient to take responsibility for his or her own health.

43. Both oral and written information should be provided. The one should not be regarded as a substitute for the other.

Patient Information Requirements

1. The purpose of the drug.
2. The effect that the drug has on the body.
3. How long it takes for the drug to act.
4. Information on the timing of the medication.
5. Information on any effect it might have on performance, eg driving.
6. Information on mixing with alcohol or other medicines.
7. Proposed duration of treatment.
8. Potential for addiction.

44. Doctors and pharmacists should ensure that patients have every opportunity to be fully informed about the risks and benefits of drug therapy. Basic education can play a significant role in motivating carers and patients to reconsider the value of drugs. Wider dissemination of information on anxiety and insomnia as normal responses to stress can reduce requests for inappropriate medication.

45. Public and professional concern about the use and misuse of benzodiazepines, viewed in terms of "risk behaviour", should be on the public health agenda. The Health Education Board for Scotland and other healthcare professionals such as district nurses, community psychiatric nurses, health visitors, hospital and community pharmacists, should be encouraged to teach the public about the rational use of benzodiazepines and promote non-drug therapies for the treatment of anxiety and insomnia.

Repeat Prescribing

46. Repeat prescribing is generally taken to mean the issue of prescriptions by general practitioners for further supplies of medication to patients on extended or long-term treatment, frequently without consultation.

47. Repeat prescribing of benzodiazepines should be an interim measure until it is possible to rationalise prescribing. Long-term prescribing cannot be eliminated quickly. Each patient on a withdrawal programme needs to be treated as an individual. This is time consuming and general practitioners can only deal with one or two patients concurrently. Long-term prescribing, and therefore repeat prescribing, is likely to decrease slowly.

48. It should be a long-term aim to remove anxiolytics and hypnotics from repeat prescribing. In the meantime, any repeat prescribing must be regularly reviewed and controlled.

49. Review mechanisms for repeat prescribing should include arrangements for regular doctor/patient consultation. Withdrawal programmes should be offered to, and agreed with, patients wherever possible. Many studies have shown that withdrawal from the therapeutic use of benzodiazepines is not always as difficult as many doctors assume and that patients, particularly those who are taking benzodiazepines intermittently, will stop when given reasons for doing so.

Review of Patients Receiving Benzodiazepines via Repeat Prescribing Systems

First, consider the purpose of the prescription. Is it -

- because there is a clinical need?

  Re-examine both the original reason and any continuing need for the treatment. Check the dose and frequency with which the drug is being taken and any medical conditions/treatment with the potential for drug interaction.

- because the patient needs to have their problem recognised with a prescription?

- because the doctor cannot resist the patient`s expectation of receiving a prescription?

Advise the patient about non-drug management, emphasising that in the long-term benzodiazepines are generally:

- not recommended
- cause drowsiness and falls
- result in psychological dependence
- reduce self-control
- reduce coping skills
- promote the sick role
- impair judgement and dexterity

Patient information leaflets reinforce the message.
Offer/negotiate a planned programme of reduction/withdrawal.

If a benzodiazepine continues to be prescribed, record each prescription issued and document:

- the advice given to the patient
- the reasons for the treatment and its proposed duration and dose (continuous or intermittent).

MANAGEMENT OF WITHDRAWAL

50. Many long-term users of benzodiazepines, anxiolytics and hypnotics who have been taking these drugs at standard doses, may be suitable candidates for a withdrawal programme.

51. Withdrawal symptoms differ according to the pharmacokinetics of the drugs involved, the daily amounts taken, the duration of use and individual sensitivity. In general terms, the risk of developing a moderate to severe withdrawal reaction is likely to be greater when the patient has been accustomed to a high dosage over a long period of time, but there is no guaranteed period of safe use.

GOOD PRACTICE IN THE MANAGEMENT OF WITHDRAWAL FROM BENZODIAZEPINES

1. The motivation of the patient is paramount. Encouragement to accept a reduction in medication should be achieved through a process of co-operation and negotiation. The goals must be simple and attainable. Patients should be left feeling that they have some control or mastery over the situation. An agreed goal should be recorded in the patient's case notes.

2. Almost any intervention can encourage some long-term users to reduce their medication. A carefully worded letter from a general practitioner can lead to between 20% and 40% of patients stopping or at least halving their intake. [Specimen letters are reproduced later in the text]

3. All patients should be assessed and counselled about their use of benzodiazepines and a timetable for gradual withdrawal established.

4. Before withdrawal is commenced, the patient should be changed onto the smallest tablet strength available of the preparation they are receiving.

5. Withdrawal should be gradual. Reductions can be calculated in steps of about 1/8 (range 1/10 $-\frac{1}{4}$) of the daily dose every fortnight.

6. Psychological support and encouragement will be needed and helps to alleviate the symptoms of withdrawal.

7. Patients who are taking a benzodiazepine other than diazepam and who are unable to reduce it, should transfer to diazepam because of its long half-life. This may also help to break the psychological dependence on the original drug.

- Transfer patient to equivalent daily dose of diazepam preferably taken at night to minimise daytime drowsiness.

- Stabilise patient before attempting withdrawal.

- Reduce diazepam dose in fortnightly steps of 2 or 2.5 mg; if withdrawal symptoms occur, maintain this dose until symptoms improve.

- Reduce dose further, if necessary, in smaller fortnightly steps; it is better to reduce too slowly rather than too quickly.

- Stop completely while some tablets remain. The time needed for withdrawal can vary from about 4 weeks to a year or more.

8. Other drugs, such as beta-blockers and buspirone, do not antagonise the benzodiazepine withdrawal syndrome and are not recommended.

9. Patients who do not respond to this type of programme, or have other complicating characteristics, should be referred to a specialist.

SUBSTITUTE DOSES OF THE COMMON BENZODIAZEPINES EXPRESSED AS DOSES OF DIAZEPAM

Chlordiazepoxide	15 mg	:	5 mg diazepam
Lorazepam	1 mg	:	10 mg diazepam
Nitrazepam	5 mg	:	5 mg diazepam
Oxazepam	15 mg	:	5 mg diazepam
Temazepam	10 mg	:	5 mg diazepam

52. Doctors and other professional workers have a leading role to fulfil in rationalising the prescribing of benzodiazepines. With their help, over 40% of patients can come off anxiolytics and hypnotics without difficulty, the next 40% may have some difficulty and the remainder may opt to remain on benzodiazepines. Any reduction is worthwhile.

SPECIMEN LETTERS

LETTER "A"

Invitation to attend for review and possible reduction of anxiolytics/hypnotics

Dear

I am writing to you because I note from our records that you have been taking .... for some time now. Recently, family doctors have become concerned about this kind of tranquillising medication when it is taken over long periods. Our concern is that the body can get used to these tablets so that they no longer work properly. If you stop taking the tablets suddenly, you may experience unpleasant withdrawal effects. For these reasons, repeated use of the tablets over a long time is no longer recommended. More importantly, these tablets may actually cause anxiety and sleeplessness and they can be addictive.

I am writing to ask you to consider cutting down on your dose of these tablets and perhaps stopping them at some time in the future. The best way to do this is to take the tablets only when you feel they are absolutely necessary. In this way you might be able to make a prescription last longer.

Once you have begun to cut down, you might be able to think about stopping them altogether. It would be best to cut down very gradually and then you will be less likely to have withdrawal symptoms.

If you would like to talk to me personally about this, I would be delighted to see you in the surgery whenever it is convenient for you to attend.

Yours sincerely

This letter may be reproduced for local use and is not bound by copyright.

LETTER "B"

To be issued when you consider that you must prescribe a benzodiazepine and to inform the patient of the reason why the prescription is short-term.

Dear

You have been prescribed ...., one of a group of medicines known as the benzodiazepines. This medicine can help you cope with a short period of severe stress; it is not intended for long-term treatment and can be habit forming.

If you are being treated for sleeplessness you will be given tablets for up to 10 nights only. Treatment for longer often makes sleep difficulties worse and may even make it difficult to stop the drug, so please do not ask for further supplies when these run out. Try to do without a sleeping tablet 1, 2 or 3 nights a week. Avoid drinks such as coffee, tea and cola after 3 pm; these contain caffeine, which can keep you awake. Avoid late-night exercise and mental stimulation.

If you are being treated for anxiety you will be given a supply of medicine for a short period.

Avoid alcoholic drinks when taking a benzodiazepine, particularly when first starting treatment.

Do not drive or operate machinery while under the effects of these drugs.

Yours sincerely

SPECIALIST REFERRAL

53. Most patients with anxiety and insomnia are managed by doctors in general practice. Indications for specialist referral are:

- Patient suitable for specialist treatment which avoids prescribing, eg behaviour or cognitive therapy.
- Failure to achieve withdrawal in certain cases after repeated treatment and advice.
- The development of severe complications of withdrawal.
- Patient simultaneously dependent on other drugs or alcohol.
- Co-existing serious physical or psychiatric morbidity.
- Patient shows signs of becoming violent.

54. The threshold for referral will be dependent upon the expertise available within the primary care team.

PROFESSIONAL EDUCATION AND TRAINING

55. Education in the range of methods for the management of anxiety and insomnia should be made available. Doctors, pharmacists, nurses, midwives and health visitors should receive basic and continuing education and training in the management of anxiety and insomnia and in the rational use of anxiolytics and hypnotics and the problems associated with their misuse. General practitioners should have courses available which are accredited for Postgraduate Education Allowance in order to update their knowledge.

AUDIT

56. Health professionals are increasingly involved in audit. Multidisciplinary audit is particularly valuable in the field of drug use and drug misuse. Scottish Prescribing Analysis (SPA) data are available to general practitioners for audit purposes and, because of their continuous availability, "before and after" studies can demonstrate changes in outcomes.

APPENDIX I

MEMBERSHIP OF WORKING GROUP

Chairman

Dr J D Gilleghan	General Practitioner Ladywell Medical Centre, Edinburgh

Members

Dr C Espie	Consultant Clinical Psychologist Arrol Park Resource Centre, Ayr
Dr G M Goodwin	MRC Clinical Scientist and Honorary Consultant Psychiatrist Medical Research Council Brain Metabolism Unit Royal Edinburgh Hospital
Mrs G T Hepburn	Pharmacist Facilitator Crosshouse Hospital
Dr I Pullen	Consultant Psychiatrist Royal Edinburgh Hospital
Dr S Ross	Medical Prescribing Adviser Ayrshire and Arran Health Board
Dr G Shirriffs	General Practitioner, Aberdeen

Officers

Mr J N Leadbeater	Administrative Secretary, SOHHD
Dr R Simmons	Medical Assessor, SOHHD
Mr I A Snedden	Assessor, Drug Misuse Branch, SOHHD

APPENDIX II

INDIVIDUALS AND ORGANISATIONS SUBMITTING EVIDENCE TO THE WORKING GROUP

Individuals:

Dr J Bury	Primary Care Facilitator, HIV/AIDS The Spittal Street Centre, Edinburgh
Dr C Freeman	Consultant Psychiatrist Royal Edinburgh Hospital
Dr J Greenwood	Consultant Psychiatrist Community Drugs Problems Service, Lothian
Dr K Mackay	Senior Registrar in Public Health Medicine Lothian Health Board
Professor I Oswald	Emeritus Professor of Psychiatry University of Edinburgh
Mr A V Stears	Home Office Drugs Inspectorate, Leeds.

Organisations:

Association of the British Pharmaceutical Industry
Association of Nurses in Substance Abuse
Centre for HIV/AIDS and Drugs Studies
Health Education Board for Scotland
Mental Health Foundation
National Nursing and Midwifery Advisory Committee
National Pharmaceutical Advisory Committee
Pharmacy Practice Division (Edinburgh)
Royal College of General Practitioners (Scottish Council)
Royal College of Psychiatrists (Scottish Division)
Scottish Association of Medical Prescribing Advisers
Scottish Drugs Forum

APPENDIX III

PHARMACOLOGY

Range of Drugs In Use for the Treatment of Anxiety and Insomnia

These are divided, for the sake of convenience, into three lists as indicated below:

Benzodiazepines available for use in the NHS	Benzodiazepines not available for use in the NHS	Other Drugs
chlordiazepoxide	alprazolam*	antidepressants-tricyclic
diazepam	bromazepam*	antidepressants-SSRI***
loprazolam	clobazam**	anti-histamines
lorazepam	clorazepate*	anti-psychotics
lormetazepam	flunitrazepam*	barbiturates
nitrazepam	flurazepam*	beta-blockers
oxazepam	medazepam*	buspirone
temazepam		chloral preparations
		chlormethiazole
		chlormezanone
		meprobamate
		monoamine-oxidase inhibitors
		zopiclone

*Drugs listed in schedule 3A to the amended NHS (General Medical and Pharmaceutical Services) Regulations, which cannot be prescribed or dispensed at NHS expense.

**NHS use restricted to epilepsy.

***SSRI = Selective Serotinin Re-uptake Inhibitor.

Indications and Choice of Medication: Benzodiazepines

1. Benzodiazepines are the most commonly used anxiolytics and hypnotics which act on receptor sites associated with gamma-aminobutyric acid (GABA) receptors. Prescribing of benzodiazepines is indicated for some non-psychological purposes, eg in the treatment of epilepsy and major muscle spasm.

2. The long-term benefits of benzodiazepines in severe illness are sometimes disputed although successful treatment without tolerance or dependence is certainly well recognised.

Common Precautions

3. Most benzodiazepines have a wide margin of safety but the following precautions should be noted:

- Benzodiazepines should not be used alone to treat depression or anxiety associated with depression because of lack of efficacy in depressive illness.
- They are not usually effective for the treatment of simple phobias or obsessional states.
- At high doses, or in susceptible individuals, and particularly in combination with alcohol, benzodiazepines may have disinhibiting effects. Aggressive behaviour towards self and others may be precipitated.
- Caution is needed when prescribing for the elderly in view of the risk of ataxia and exacerbation or induction of mental confusion.
- Patients with known respiratory problems, or where there is evidence of respiratory interruption during sleep (sleep apnoea) should not be prescribed hypnotic drugs.
- Caution should be taken in prescribing benzodiazepines to patients with hepatic or renal impairment since they may cause encephalopathy.
- Caution should be exercised when prescribing benzodiazepines during pregnancy, especially during the first trimester, but also during the last trimester, since the drugs enter the foetal circulation and can lead to loss of

muscle tone, feeding difficulties and a withdrawal syndrome in the newborn. Benzodiazepines should not be prescribed for breast feeding mothers because of the risk of accumulation in the infant.

Interaction with other Medicines

4. Benzodiazepines may enhance the sedative effects of alcohol, anaesthetics, antidepressants, antihistamines and antipsychotics. They may also enhance the hypotensive effect of antihypertensives. Cimetidine may enhance the effect of benzodiazepines because it inhibits their metabolism.

Side Effects during Treatment with Benzodiazepines

5. The most common side effect during treatment is daytime drowsiness which is hazardous for drivers or those operating machinery, even if not obvious. Other adverse effects include ataxia, difficulty with balance, anterograde amnesia and impaired concentration. These effects are dose related and cease when the drug is eliminated from the body.

Duration of Action of Benzodiazepines

6. Short-acting benzodiazepines are preferred for hypnotic use since otherwise unwanted sedative effects persist on the morning after taking the drug. Longer acting drugs are more appropriate for anxiety states but their sedative effects may build up in proportion to the accumulation of the drug in the body.

Withdrawal from Benzodiazepines

7. Withdrawal is characterised by anxiety, insomnia, tremor, tachycardia, loss of appetite and excessive sensitivity to light and sound. Epileptic seizures and psychotic phenomena may also occur, but are rare. All the common symptoms may be seen in the original illness but the perceptual changes are characteristic of the withdrawal syndrome.

8. These symptoms can occur following therapeutic doses given for short periods of time (3-14 days) but they are generally mild and not everyone experiences them. They are commoner in people with dependent personality traits. Withdrawal symptoms usually appear shortly after abruptly stopping a benzodiazepine with a short half-life, or up to several days after stopping one with a long half-life. The

rebound phenomena are not related to the length of prescribing, nor to the particular drug prescribed. Some individuals report long-term difficulties after stopping benzodiazepines but the balance of causes in such cases is often open to different interpretations.

Psychological Factors

9. Some patients can become psychologically dependent upon taking medication. This can contribute to problems upon withdrawal, but does not account for the existence of the withdrawal syndrome.

Tolerance

10. Despite some evidence to the contrary, the UK Committee on the Review of Medicines has concluded that hypnotic drugs are not effective over long periods of continuous use and that the pharmacodynamic effectiveness of anxiolytic drugs is reduced after 4 months continuous treatment. This is an area that requires critical re-assessment in future studies.

Effect of Higher Doses

11. There is very little evidence to suggest that the administration of higher doses of benzodiazepines is justifiable. Higher doses are more likely to produce intoxication in the short-term and tolerance in the long-term. For example, a daily dose of 20-30 mgs of diazepam should be regarded as a maximum. Requests for higher doses from patients is prima facie evidence for drug misuse.

Toxicity in Overdose

12. Although benzodiazepines are much safer in overdose than, for example, barbiturates, they have the potential to interact with other drugs and alcohol, and their misuse is a contributory cause of many deaths. In the case of accidental overdosage or deliberate self-poisoning, careful management, with reference to an emergency protocol, is particularly indicated in the elderly, patients with chronic pulmonary disease and in all circumstances where overdosage is combined with other central nervous system (CNS) depressant agents.

Indications and Choice of Medication: Other Drugs

13. Tricyclic antidepressants are effective in anxiety, panic and phobic disorders but there is a risk of relapse when the drugs are withdrawn. They are more toxic than benzodiazepines in overdose.

14. SSRI antidepressants appear to be effective in panic disorder and also obsessional compulsive disorder where anxiety symptoms are also prominent. They do not have a defined role in the management of mild anxiety states although they may have the potential, like tricyclics, to cover benzodiazepine withdrawal. This requires further study.

15. Antihistamines are sometimes used as hypnotics in paediatric or geriatric practice.

16. Antipsychotics have been used in low dosages but are associated with a risk of movement disorder which may be permanent.

17. Barbiturates are effective hypnotics but have unacceptable risks of dependency, and toxicity in overdose.

18. In general, beta-blockers have no direct effect on psychological symptoms and are only effective in patients with somatic symptoms, usually with performance anxiety. Propranolol crosses the blood brain barrier and causes significant central nervous system side effects in some people. There is a risk of inducing asthma in susceptible individuals.

19. Buspirone is a newer drug which is thought to act at specific serotonin receptors rather than the GABA receptors. Its dependence potential has not been established and it is not a drug which appears to be currently misused.

20. Chloral derivatives such as chloral hydrate and chloral betaine can be used for the treatment of insomnia but carry a risk of gastric irritation, can lead to dependence because they are structurally related to alcohol, and are dangerous in overdose.

21. Chlormethiazole has both hypnotic and anticonvulsant properties. It has a short half life and may cause less confusion in the elderly than benzodiazepines. It

has a pharmacology related to barbiturates and the benzodiazepines, is a drug of misuse, and is dangerous in overdose.

22. Meprobamate is less effective than a benzodiazepine, carries greater risk in overdose and can also induce dependence.

23. Monoamine-oxidase inhibitors are sometimes used in severe anxiety states by psychiatrists. The older drugs are non-selective and irreversible which means that they require dietary precautions and are dangerous in overdose. Reversible inhibitors of monoamine-oxidase inhibitors (RIMAs), such as moclobemide, have been introduced recently and may come to play a role in the treatment of severe anxiety states.

24. Zopiclone is not a benzodiazepine but acts on a related domain of the GABA receptor. Its pharmacology is sufficiently like that of the benzodiazepines to raise the suspicion that it is likely to have similar disadvantages. It remains to be established that it does not cause dependence and problems on withdrawal.

APPENDIX IV

SOURCES OF INFORMATION AND ADVICE

The British National Formulary

1. The British National Formulary (BNF), which offers advice on the properties of drugs, dosages, generic equivalents, side-effects, drug interactions and guidelines on withdrawal, is generally regarded as the benchmark of good prescribing practice. It is updated every six months.

General Practice Formularies

2. Many general practices have produced their own general practice formularies and, as a result of discussions with pharmacists and clinical pharmacologists, it is likely that many practices have already made policy decisions on the prescribing of benzodiazepines.

Medical Prescribing Advisers

3. Medical prescribing advisers (MPAs) are employed by Health Boards. Their remit is to liaise between Health Board managers, practices and individual general practitioners on prescribing matters and to offer advice on good prescribing policy. They are expected to acquire a thorough knowledge of the different practices in their area and are therefore in an informed position to offer relevant and helpful advice. Medical prescribing advisers are keen to help general practitioners who are experiencing difficulties related to prescribing benzodiazepines and other drugs.

Psychiatric Advice

4. Psychiatrists with an interest in general practitioner liaison and the management of anxiety, insomnia, and drug misuse, can provide specialist advice.

Clinical Psychology Advice

5. Clinical psychologists are often willing to act on a consultancy basis with practices to provide advice on strategies for managing potentially large numbers of patients with anxiety and sleep problems. This can facilitate the selective direct referral of more severe or complex problems for individual therapy.

Drug and Therapeutics Committees

6. These committees, which exist at Area and Unit level and also within NHS Trusts, initiate and co-ordinate drug policies and prepare prescribing guidelines for use in the hospital and the community. They also provide a valuable forum for the discussion of problems at the interface between primary and secondary care.

Hospital Pharmacists

7. Ward-based clinical pharmacists are in a key position to influence prescribing practice through involvement in the preparation of prescribing protocols, prescription monitoring, drug history taking and related activities. They also provide a drug information service which is available to all healthcare staff.

Pharmaceutical Prescribing Advisers

8. Pharmaceutical prescribing advisers work directly with community pharmacists and general practitioners by invitation. They can provide advice aimed at encouraging rational prescribing, for example, the development, use and monitoring of general practice policies or formularies, the analysis of prescribing data, or help with audit.

Community Pharmacists

9. The Community pharmacist is an important source of professional expertise and advice and is well placed to counsel patients on the administration and storage of medicines as well as giving advice on general health matters. Time should be set aside for counselling all patients in receipt of benzodiazepines. Community pharmacies can serve as a useful focus for health education activities and the dissemination of patient leaflets. It is essential that pharmacists and general practitioners develop shared aims in the management of benzodiazepine abuse, so that the message coming from the general practitioner is reinforced by the pharmacist.

Drug Information Service

10. At Health Board level, all Boards have, or have access to, a drug information service which can provide expert advice to doctors and pharmacists in response to individual enquiries. Prescribers are encouraged to make contact with their local Drug Information Centre.

Common Services Agency

11. The Common Services Agency provides a range of information services:

- Viewdata Information Services contains comprehensive information on drugs and provides up-to-date comparative information on costs. This information, which is stored on computer, can be accessed using a microcomputer linked to the main computer via a modem.

- The Scottish Medicines Resource Centre produces regular bulletins on evaluated drug information for general practitioners.

- The Pharmacy Practice Division provides information on medicine usage and costs to all general practitioners using Scottish Prescription Analysis data (SPA).

12. Whilst prescription numbers do not give an accurate reflection of the total quantities prescribed and offer no indication of strength, the use of defined daily doses as a research tool provides a useful mechanism for determining the overall usage of a particular drug and allows comparison of drug consumption between practices and health boards.

APPENDIX V

CONTROLLING FACTORS

1. The principal legislation concerned with the control of drugs in the United Kingdom is the Misuse of Drugs Act 1971 and its associated legislation. Most benzodiazepines are classified under Schedule 4 of the Misuse of Drugs Regulations 1985 and therefore come under the control of the 1971 Act. However, they are not notifiable drugs and they are not subject to the full range of restrictions which apply to controlled drugs, including safe custody and registers. It is a current concern that prescribed benzodiazepines may find their way on to the illicit market because patients sell them on or some doctors may over-prescribe to misusers themselves.

2. The Home Office Drugs Inspectorate, which is responsible for supervising the legitimate production and distribution of controlled drugs, is also responsible for investigating cases of suspected irresponsible prescribing. In practice, the limited resources of the Home Office Drugs Inspectorate makes prompt intervention difficult. There is less information concerning "lower schedule" controlled drugs than for Schedule 2 drugs. To date, no Scottish case of drug misuse has been referred to a Misuse of Drugs Tribunal, but prescribers must always be prepared to justify the use of benzodiazepines on clinical grounds.

3. Any cases of apparently excessive prescribing by general medical practitioners identified by the Pharmacy Practice Division on cost grounds, or by other sources, (eg the police), on other grounds, are investigated by the Medical Prescribing Adviser of the appropriate Health Board who will usually be able to deal with the matter informally. Otherwise, the Health Board may seek the opinion of the Area Medical Committee, which has powers to investigate such matters. On receipt of all the information, the Health Board makes a decision on action, and there is a right of appeal to the Secretary of State.

4. The role of the doctor as a professional is very important in controlling misuse.

All benzodiazepines are prescription only medicines (POMs), ie they can only legally be obtained on prescription. The need for good prescribing practice is clear, and general practitioners are aware of the dangers of dependence on these drugs. The British National Formulary, which is issued by the Health Departments to all doctors, has for some years contained warnings against treatment with benzodiazepines for extended periods of time. The Committee on Safety of Medicines has also sent advice to all doctors emphasising strongly the dangers of dependence on benzodiazepines, and has advised doctors to limit their use to the short-term relief of severe anxiety or insomnia.

5. Locally agreed voluntary bans on the prescribing of certain benzodiazepines have been introduced in a number of Health Board areas in an attempt to reduce the prevalence of misuse.

APPENDIX VI

DRUG MISUSE

1. By the end of the 1980s, there was extensive misuse of benzodiazepines, both orally and by injection, among young poly-drug misusers in Scotland. Misuse is most prevalent in the cities and larger conurbations but it is also prevalent in the more rural areas of Scotland. The number of misusers and the drug of misuse reported is shown in Table III which indicates that temazepam is the drug most misused in Scotland when "Temazepam - other" and "Temazepam - prescribed only" are added together. Heroin and buprenorphine are the drugs most likely to be injected (80% and 76% respectively). The proportion of all those reporting temazepam use who were injecting the drug is 26% (34% for 1991/92). When prescribed temazepam is excluded, the percentage injecting the drug rises to 32%.

2. The most popular benzodiazepine preparation for misuse is the 20mg temazepam gel-filled capsule. It is believed that in Glasgow this drug is misused by as many as 50% of illicit intravenous drug users on a daily basis. Other strengths of temazepam capsules, temazepam tablets and various solid dose formulations of diazepam are also popular.

3. The level of reported thefts from producers, wholesalers and pharmacies is believed to be small. There is evidence from the Home Office Drugs Inspectorate that the vast majority of misused benzodiazepines are obtained on prescription. Information suggests that it is common practice in some areas for therapeutic supplies of benzodiazepines prescribed in good faith to be made available to misusers. In some cases the person to whom the drug has been prescribed sees the opportunity for financial gain, while in others, the patient is intimidated into handing over the drugs or the prescription. Anecdotal reports exist of persons travelling outside their normal areas of residence to register with general practitioners in order to obtain supplies to sell to a third party. Misusers or their associates appear to be able to obtain prescriptions on the basis of stated, feigned or exaggerated clinical symptoms with relative ease.

4. It is rarely possible to predict accurately what impact specific control measures will have on drug misuse. For example, the decrease in the supply of heroin in Scotland in the mid eighties did not lead to a reduction in drug usage, but resulted instead in a shift to the misuse of pharmaceutical drugs. Similarly, with regard to temazepam, replacement of the liquid-filled capsule with the gel-filled capsule failed to prevent drug misusers from injecting the contents, with catastrophic consequences of limb amputations. There is no simple solution to this problem, and general practitioners must be vigilant at all times when deciding whether or not to prescribe a benzodiazepine to a patient, particularly one who is temporarily registered or one who is a known drug misuser.

5. Experience suggests that it is relatively easy to support drug misusers to reduce the amount of benzodiazepines that they are taking from levels of, for example, 40-50 mgs of diazepam and 60 mgs of temazepam to doses at the top of the therapeutic range. Reduction from maximum recommended doses to complete withdrawal seems to be much more difficult for all types of patients.

6. The "Good Practice in the Management of Withdrawal of Benzodiazepines" Guide (located between paragraphs 51 and 52) is applicable to withdrawal in drug misusers. However, the social and psychological problems of young polydrug misusers are likely to be very different from those of other patients who are dependent upon benzodiazepines alone. Specialist services, such as Community Drugs Problems Services, should be available to assist in the management of more difficult cases on a shared care basis.

TABLE III: ALL DRUGS OF MISUSE REPORTED TO THE SCOTTISH DRUG MISUSE DATABASE

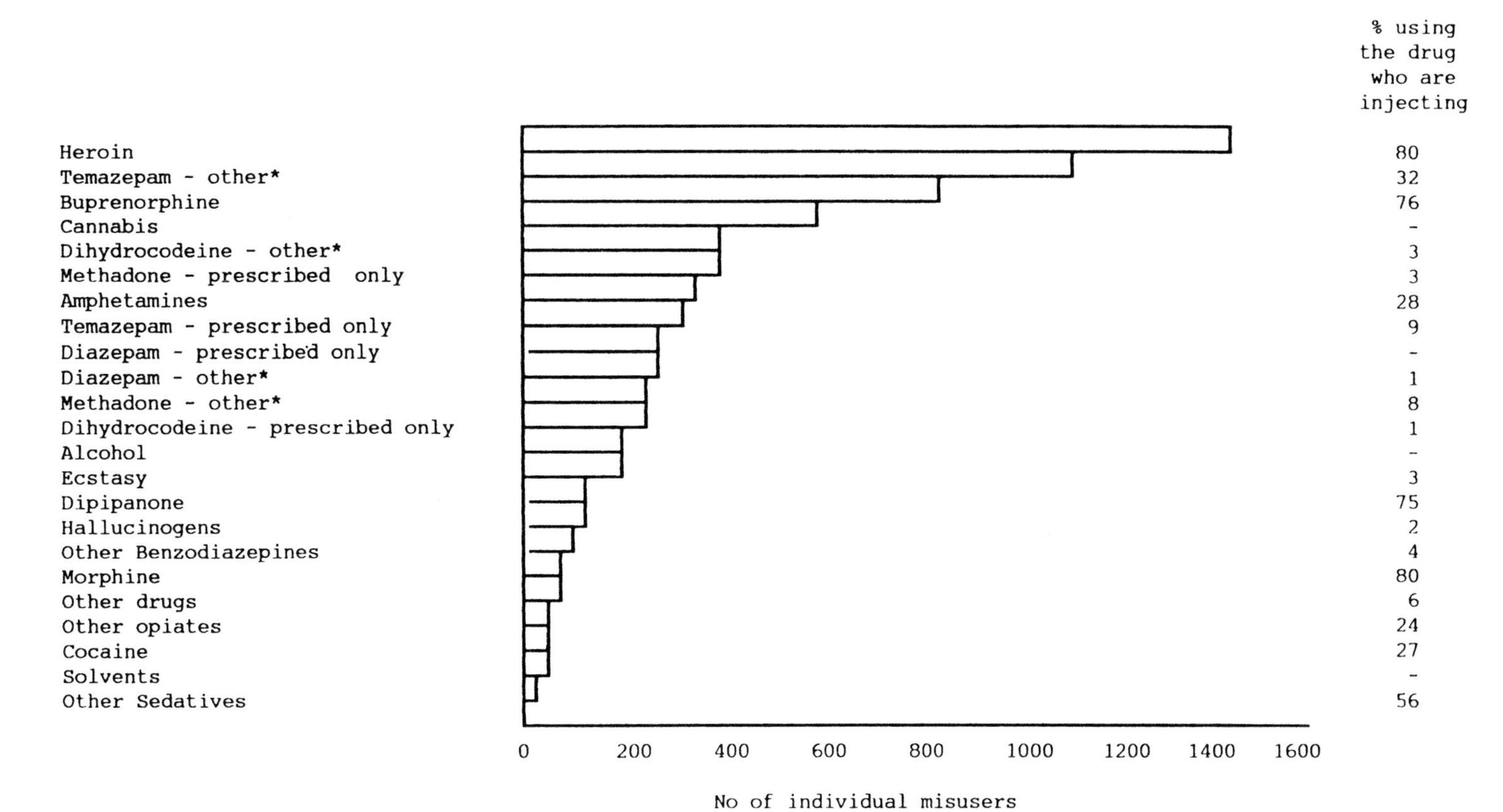

*"other" refers to instances where some or all of the drugs are obtained illicitly or the source is unknown.

Source: Scottish Drug Misuse Database Bulletin, 1993. Information and Statistics Division, Scottish Health Service Common Services Agency.

APPENDIX VII

RECOMMENDED READING

Drug Misuse and Dependence - Guidelines on Clinical Management. Department of Health, Scottish Office Home and Health Department, Welsh Office. London, HMSO, 1991.

Benzodiazepines, Dependence and Withdrawal Symptoms.
Committee on Safety of Medicines. Current Problems No 21, 1988.

Russell J, Lader M (eds). Guidelines for the Prevention and Treatment of Benzodiazepine Dependence. Mental Health Foundation, 1993.

Benzodiazepines: The Problem of Misuse and Dependence. Welsh Committee on Drug Misuse, 1991.

Haw S, Pharmaceutical Drugs and Illicit Drug Use in Lothian Region. Centre for HIV/AIDS and Drugs Studies (CHADS), 1993.

Shapiro C M (ed). ABC of Sleep Disorders, BMJ Publishing Group, London, 1993.

Gudex C. Adverse Effects of Benzodiazepines. University of York. Centre for Health Economics, Health Economics Consortium Discussion Paper 65, 1990.

Cormack M A et al. Evaluation of an easy, cost-effective strategy for cutting benzodiazepine use in general practice. *British Journal of General Practice* 1994, 44. 5-8.

NATIONAL MEDICAL ADVISORY COMMITTEE

The National Medical Advisory Committee provides medical advice to the Scottish Office Home and Health Department and to the Chief Medical Officer for Scotland.

PUBLICATIONS

Diagnostic and Interventional Radiology in Scotland - Into the Nineties	(1990)
Neonatal Care in Scotland	(1990)
The Future of Mental Handicap Hospital Services in Scotland	(1992)
Infertility Services in Scotland	(1993)
Rehabilitation Services in Scotland	(1993)
The Management of Patients with Stroke	(1993)
Vascular Surgery Services in Scotland	(1994)
The Management of Patients with Chronic Pain	(1994)
The Management of Anxiety and Insomnia	(1994)

These publications may be obtained from HMSO bookshops or their accredited agents.

Printed for HMSO Scotland Dd.0293070 10/94